Rejuvenation and Life Extension
Secrets to a Long and Healthy Life Full of Vitality

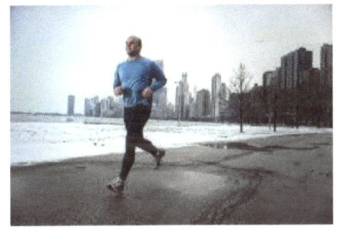

Introduction

Each one of us has the desire of having a long, healthy life. The good news is that with a bit of planning and by including certain restrictions in our daily life we can achieve that easily. In this book, I have discussed a series of useful rejuvenation and life extension techniques. Incorporate them into your life to live longer and enjoy your life more.

Chapter 1
How to Rejuvenate Your System?

Before introducing you to different methods of rejuvenating your system, I would like you to know what the term "rejuvenation" actually means. It's a discipline that focuses on practical reversal of the aging process. You shouldn't confuse rejuvenation with life extension. It's because Life extension typically involves studying the factors that trigger aging and opposing them with the aim of slowing down the aging process. Now, read on to know how to rejuvenate your system.

Rejuvenation Techniques You Can Try

Boost the thyroid gland- When we start growing older, our thyroid gland stops functioning properly. This happens because of iodine deficiency. Iodine plays an extremely important role in the process of metabolism. We need this nutrient for healthy nerve and muscle function and adequate production of blood cells. In addition, iodine is also essential for having healthy nails, teeth and skin.

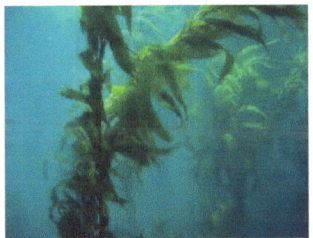

To boost your thyroid function, you can add iodine-rich food items such as kelp, dulse (they are both seaweeds) etc. to your daily diet. In addition, make sure that you are only having iodized salt.

Practice yoga- Yoga is known for having amazing anti-aging benefits. There are a number of yoga asanas that can help you to reverse your aging process, but the one that's known to be most effective is the Salamba Sarvangasana or the Shoulder Stand. This yoga posture rejuvenates our system by improving our thyroid functions. Find out how to perform Salamba Sarvangasana.

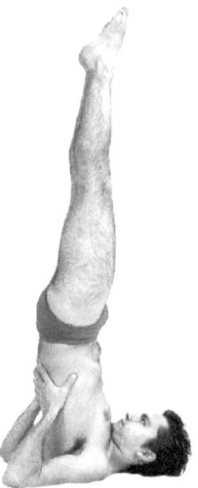

1. Lie down with your back on the yoga mat. Keep the legs together.
2. Start raising your legs towards the ceiling. Continue until your legs form an angle of 90 degrees with your neck/shoulders.
3. Now, with your chin tucked in your chest, rest your entire body weight on your elbows and shoulders. While doing so, you should use your arms for supporting your hips.
4. When in this position, you shouldn't look sideways as that might hurt your back and neck badly.

Perform breathing exercises-

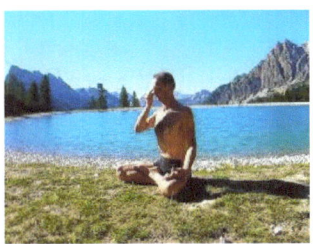

Performing breathing exercise would promote rejuvenation and relaxation of your body and mind. You will see your mind developing more clarity and there will also be a significant increase in your sense of wellbeing. Breathing exercises work by promoting deep inhalations, which allows our body to receive increased amount of oxygen.

Sleep well- As we age, we tend to lose our ability to fall asleep easily. Many of us also suffer from sleep deprivation. However, the fact is that lack of sound sleep is one of the main causes of several age-related disorders. So, to make sure that we have a healthy old age, we must take steps for improving our sleep pattern. An effective way of promoting sound sleep is unwinding for a minimum of one hour before going to bed. This can be done either by meditating, praying or just by lying on the bed and doing nothing. These actions help in releasing the stress we gathered during the rest of the day allowing us to sleep properly.

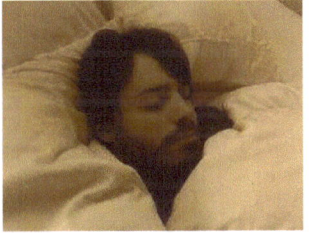

Having a good night's sleep is essential for looking young and radiant. When we sleep, our cells get repaired and our body releases a couple of essential hormones, melatonin and human growth hormone or HGH. These are the hormones responsible for promoting youthfulness. Other than improving our skin condition and rejuvenating body, these hormones also boost our immune system.

Try herbal remedies- There are certain herbs that have amazing anti-aging benefits. Use them for getting rid of various symptoms of aging. Below are some herbs you can try.

- **Parsley-**

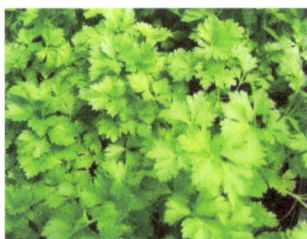

    Parsley, which is a rich source of pro-vitamin V, vitamin C and chlorophyll, is known for its skin cleansing, soothing and stimulating properties. To experience these benefits of the herb, you should drink an infusion prepared using it once or twice everyday day. Applying the infusion on your face is also highly beneficial, particularly for individuals suffering from age-related skin problems. Regular consumption of the infusion is also known for boosting the thyroid gland, liver, lungs, bladder, kidney and stomach.

- **Schizandra-**

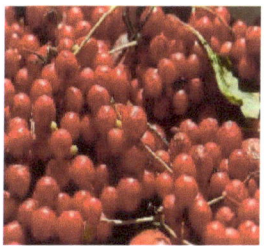

When consumed in reasonable amount this herb works as an energy booster, which rejuvenates our entire system. If you take schizandra regularly, you will see significant improvement in your ability to exercise.

- **Gotu kola-**

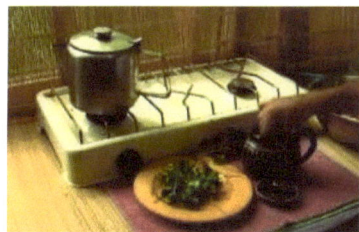

Lack of mental clarity is a problem most elderly individual face. Gotu kola would be a great herbal remedy for them. It is capable of improving mental clarity and alleviating anxiety. Ideally, you should consume this herb in form of an herbal infusion.

- **Gynostema-**

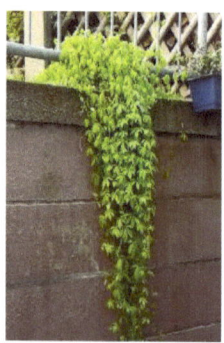

If you are suffering from lack of stamina due to old age, I would suggest you to consume gynostema regularly. It works by improving our mental balance and increasing our stamina. The herb also promotes the functioning of our nervous and immune system.

- **Siberian ginseng-**

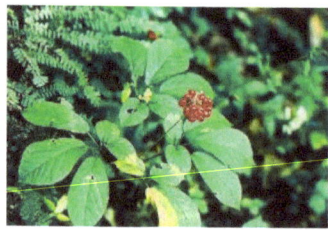

This is another herb that can increase your energy and vitality. You will get this herb both in form of capsules and powder. Use the powdered Siberian ginseng for preparing an aromatic tea. Drinking the tea twice daily will allow aging individuals to complete their daily jobs with the same vigor as a 25 year old.

- **Astragalus-**

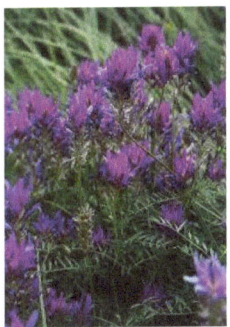

Other than being a highly effective energy booster, this herb also helps in boosting our appetite and eliminating weakness, both of which are problems associated with increasing age. Astragalus also improves our ability to fight diseases.

Practice detox bath- Toxins accumulated in different organs and tissues of our body stimulate the aging process. Thus to rejuvenate our system, it's extremely important that we get rid of those toxins. The best way of doing that is practicing detox bath. Detox bath works by regenerating our body. You will see your skin becoming tighter, hair turning thicker and stronger and body becoming more toned. In addition, the action of this bath on our root chakra helps in boosting sexual function and libido naturally. It's a known fact that being sexually active is one of the most effective anti-aging techniques. Below I have described the process of a couple of detox baths.

- **Epsom salt bath-**

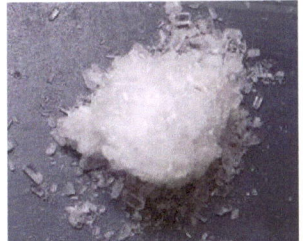

Detoxifying baths using Epsom salts (Hydrated Magnesium Sulfate) enjoys significant popularity all around the globe. The main reasons behind this are the low cost and easy availability of Epsom salts. This detoxifying bath works by replenishing the magnesium reserves in our system and eliminating the accumulated toxins from our organs. Here, it must be noted that magnesium, which is an alkaline mineral, holds the 4th spot in the list of essential minerals in human body. Magnesium deficiency has become extremely common these days due to poor lifestyle and bad dietary habits. Practicing Epsom salt bath regularly will offer you the following benefits.

- Boost circulation
- Ease hypertension
- Improve oxygen use
- Reduce inflammation
- Encourage mineral use

Here are the steps of Epsom salt bath:

- Take two cup of Epsom salts (you can also use a combination of Epsom salts, apple cider vinegar, baking soda or your favorite essential oils).
- Put the Epsom salts into your bathtub and dilute them in hot water. If you want, add a few drops of tea tree, lavender, or rose essential oil to the mix and allow the ingredients to soak for 30 to 40 minutes.
- The water is now ready for being used for a perfect detox bath. The water should just be lukewarm when you use it for bathing.

- **Ginger detox bath-**

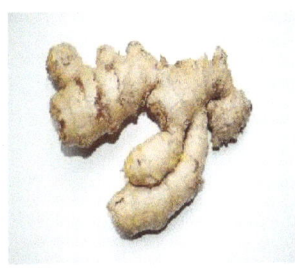

Ginger bath helps in releasing all the toxins stored in our body in form of sweat. Since the ancient times, sweating has been one of the most widely used methods of eliminating impurities and toxins from their body and maintaining good health. You can experience similar benefits by practicing ginger bath regularly.

Here are the steps of ginger bath:

- For this recipe, you will either need ginger powder or freshly grated ginger. Add a teaspoonful of ginger powder or half a cup of grated ginger to hot water.
- Allow the ingredient to soak for 20 to 30 minutes. Once the water is lukewarm, take the bath.

Ginger bath will result in profuse sweating. You will be sweating even after an hour of taking the bath. So, don't wear your regular clothing immediately after bathing. Instead, wear sweat clothes or your bathrobe.

Also, to prevent dehydration, you should drink plenty of water after taking this detox bath. Allergy prone individuals should taste ginger on their skin to check whether they are allergic to it before they proceed.

Chapter 2
Life Extension Tips and Techniques

The term "life extension" is used for the study of reversing or slowing down the aging process for extending both average and maximum lifespan. It works by spotting the factors responsible for aging and then fights them to stop the aging process.

Life extension techniques you can try

- One of the most widely used techniques of life extension is taking steps for preventing the most common causes of death. It involves taking care of an individual's brain and heart health, making him/her undergo regular cancer screening and so on.

- Another common method is keeping the level of different natural chemicals produced within our body including hormones similar to what we find in a twenty year old. Several studies conducted over the years have also shown that on many occasions decline in the level of natural chemicals is not just the effect, but the cause of the onset of the process of aging.

    o One hormone that has direct link with our aging process is the growth hormone (HGH). Decline in the levels of HGH can be managed using hormone replacement therapy. However, that method is mostly used just for slowing down the aging process in people over 40. If you are under 40, experts might use growth hormone releasing substances for stimulating production of HGH naturally. I have discussed HGH and its impact on life extension in detail later in this chapter.

    o Two other hormones that play vital roles in life extension are pregnenolone and dehydroepiandrosterone (DHEA). The market is filled with supplements with pregnenolone and DHEA as their main ingredients. However, you must be cautious when using those supplements as overconsumption of DHEA might make you suffer from serious side effects. For best results, take those supplements under the supervision of a medical practitioner.

- Aging leads to a significant drop in the level of the neurotransmitter dopamine. This happens primarily because of the rise in the levels of another brain chemical called MAO-B or type B monoamine oxidase. MAO-B works by destroying dopamine and many other neuro-chemicals. This problem can be managed through administration of low doses of deprenyl. It's a prescription drug that works by inhibiting MAO-B's activity and boosting the levels of dopamine. In addition, when taken in cognition with antioxidants, deprenyl can offer protection to critical brain cells against damage.

- Aging can be triggered by loss of insulin sensitivity, a condition that causes unstable and high levels of blood sugar. These changes in our system start damaging vital proteins, which affect our organs, skin and hair badly. This makes treating insulin sensitivity one of the most widely used life extension techniques.

- The aging process often makes us suffer from sleep deprivation. This happens primarily due to the decrease in production of melatonin, a hormone responsible for controlling our sleep and wake cycles.

  Many scientists believe that melatonin play the role of master hormone when it comes to aging. This means melatonin signals other hormones to speed up the process of aging. As a result, life extension often involves replacement of melatonin orally.

* Intake of vitamin C supplements is another commonly used life expectancy technique. The concept was introduced by Nobel laureate

Dr. Linus Pauling. He himself began taking high dosages of the vitamin in 1965. Pauling had a long life and died in 1994 when he was 93. According to Pauling, he could delay his death by almost two decades just because of the vitamin C supplements he consumed. During the final years of his life, he used to take as much as 18,000 mg of the vitamin every day. His study on Vitamin C, on the other hand, suggested that if one takes 3,200-12,000 mg of the vitamin per day, he/she can expect to live for an additional 12 to 18 years. I would, however, suggest you not to follow these suggestions without consulting a doctor. It's because overconsumption of the vitamin might lead to toxicity.

Vitamin C is water soluble and is not produced naturally in our body. As a result, for enabling life extension through this vitamin we would need to consume fruits and vegetables rich in vitamin C. Examples of food items rich in vitamin C are Brussels sprouts, citrus fruits, tomatoes, papaya etc. You can also consume vitamin C supplement.

You will also get vitamin C in fat-soluble form. It's called ascorbyl palmitate. Findings of Dr. Pauling's study revealed that once ascorbyl palmitate is absorbed, it fortifies our blood vessels' micro-capillary walls, which often get damaged as we grow old. Pauling's study also found that when consumed along with amino acids such as L-proline and L-lysine, vitamin C can reduce atherosclerosis plagues substantially.

Some experts also recommend consumption of vitamin D for life extension. It's probably because studies conducted in recent times have revealed that supplementation of this vitamin can slow down the aging process and prevent cancer and heart disease, two of the most common causes of death globally.

Recently, a group of scientists found that D3, the precursor of vitamin D is present is several other tissues besides the bone. For instance, our skin has a high percentage of D3. This makes the role of this vitamin in life extension more important.

Life extension by optimizing levels of human growth hormone (HGH)

Individuals looking to increase endogenous production of HGH can be benefited hugely by effective nutritional strategies. The nutrients used for this purpose works either by increasing the efficacy of exercise or sleep (these two activities are known to have biggest impact on the production of HGH) or by increasing HGH release from our pituitary gland.

A compound called cytidine-5-diposphate choline or CDP-choline has been found to boost production of HGH while improving the brain health of aging adults. Increase in age often hampers production of HGH from our anterior pituitary significantly. According to a recent study, this decrease in secretion of HGH is partly due to increase in the production of somatostatin. This finding forced researchers to look for substances that can inhibit production of somatostatin and thereby increase GHG secretion.

After carrying out a series of experiments, they came to know that cholinergic agonists are capable of increasing HGH production by slowing down release of somatostatin from our hypothalamus. Soon, these findings were even supported by evidence gathered during a human study. When treated with CDP-choline, healthy elderly individuals experienced a dramatic increase in their HGH levels.

That's not all. CDP-choline was also found to be highly effective in promoting brain cell health and integrity in elderly people. This agent plays the role of a mediator in the formation of the neuronal membranes. This ensures healthy brain cell functions and proper brain cell membrane structure.

Clinical trials conducted using CDP-choline showed that the agent might be useful in reversing age-related memory impairment. It works by counteracting amyloid-beta deposition. This pathological protein is one of the biggest indicators of Alzheimer's disease. A recently conducted human research revealed that CDP-choline has a vital role to play even in the secretion of neurotransmitter norepinephrine. The agent has also been found to possess the ability of supporting recovery from two of the most common causes of death, hemorrhagic and ischemic strokes.

Proteins, particularly those extracted from animals, are rich sources of essential amino acids known for their ability of assisting production of HGH. In addition, these amino acids also play vital roles in the process of muscle recovery and growth in active women and men. The amino acid that is found most abundantly in human body is glutamine. Glutamine has shown amazing results in increasing HGH levels even when consumed in a very small amount (2,000 mg). This amino acid also possess the ability to protect muscle mass of people susceptible to muscle loss due to surgery-induced inactivity.

Another amino acid that can play a significant role in life extension is arginine. Oral consumption of arginine-based nutritional supplements can increase GH production at rest. If you exercise regularly when taking arginine supplement, the results will be even better.

HGH production can also be increased through consumption of ornithine alpha-ketoglutarate, an agent primarily known for its anabolic effects. Studies have shown that arginine, when consumed in cognition with ornithine alpha-ketoglutarate, makes the process developing muscle strength and lean muscle mass much easier by augmenting the effects of resistance training. Here, it must be mentioned that for most people daily consumption of 1 gm of ornithine alpha-ketoglutarate is enough.

Chapter 3
About Sperm Building Techniques

One of the most common purposes of practicing life extension techniques is maintaining vitality and sperm health. This chapter will educate you about different sperm building technique and dietary habits that can help you to have healthier sperm count.

Techniques for boosting sperm production

Bee pollen

Bee pollen, due to its natural ability of fertilizing, is widely used for stimulating sperm production. More than twenty studies conducted in recent times have found that sexual health of men can be improved dramatically using bee pollen. A recently published German study revealed that men suffering from prostate problem, a common age-related disorder, can be benefited significantly by this natural ingredient. According to the findings of the study, supplementation of bee pollen decreased prostate pain and increased sexual pleasure in people taking part in the study.

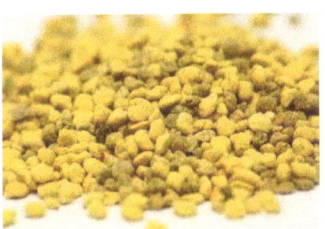

Individuals with chronic prostate problems experience buildup of free radicals in their seminal fluid. These free radicals result in burns at cellular levels. Bee pollen works by easing such burnings and thereby allows men with prostate disorders enjoy intimacy with their partner without experiencing any swelling or burning sensation.

Studies conducted in China revealed that male infertility and chronic prostate inflammation are both results of free radical buildup. Researchers carrying out those studies tested several agents that were found to possess the ability of destroying and stopping formation of the free radicals. They found that bee pollen offered the best results.

Supplementation of bee pollen not only increase fertility and sperm count, but also allows sperm to swim faster and last longer. Other than being a highly powerful antioxidant, this natural agent is also a rich source of zinc, a mineral known for its natural libido boosting qualities.

Carotenes

Carotenes like lycopene, lutein and beta-carotene play big roles in overall maintenance of human health. Now, a new study has revealed that lutein and beta-carotene are capable of promoting better sperm movement. Consumption of lycopene, on the other hand, has been found to improve shape and size of sperms. The study was carried out on men who are still at the university. Researchers chose men of this age group for their study as they wanted to show the world that sperm quality and morphology are in decline even in men who should have the healthiest sperm. This highlights the importance of taking care of sperm quality in older men. Since a long time, women have been using nutritional supplements for enhancing their prenatal health. This new study shows that doing something similar is important even for the men.

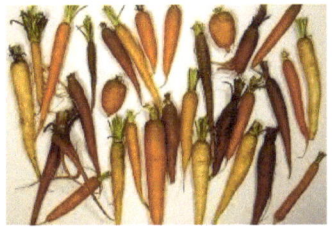

The lycopene or beta carotene supplements men take for improving their sperm health should always be 100% natural. Read the label of the products carefully to gather knowledge about the sources of the ingredients before consuming the supplements.

Folic acid

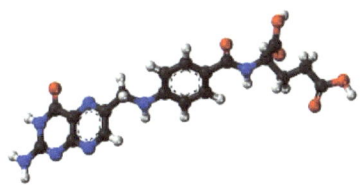

Men with folic acid deficiency tend to have lower sperm count. Supplementation of folic acid has been found to significantly reduce the occurrence of sperm disorders in healthy men. Consumption of 400 micrograms of folic acid per day is enough for bringing back your sperm count to normal. Some food sources of this nutrient are orange juice, legumes, leafy greens, breakfast cereals etc. Consuming a glassful of orange juice 20 to 30 minutes before intimacy has been found to increase sperm count drastically. You can also take folic acid supplements under medical supervision.

L-arginine

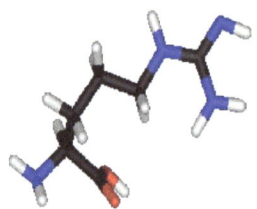

This nutrient plays an important role in production, and maturation of sperm. Supplementation of this nutrient is known to increase sperm count and enhance motility and quality of sperms. However, here, it must be noted that you will not be benefited much if your initial sperm count is less than 10million/ml. Men suffering from sperm abnormalities are often advised to take 500 mg L-arginine every day. However, the maximum dose of L-arginine prescribed by doctors is 4 grams per day.

L-carnitine

This nutrient enables proper maturation of sperms and ensures that they function properly. L-carnitine is secreted by our epididymis. The anti-oxidants present in this nutrient protect sperms form damages caused by free radicals. According to health practitioners, a daily dose of 1 to 2 mg L-carnitine is enough for increasing motility, and quality of sperm in men with sperm abnormalities.

Food items you should include in your daily diet to improve your sperm quality

Eggs-

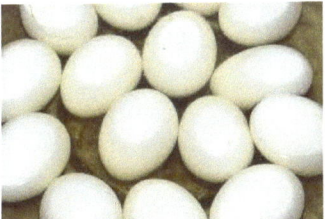

The high levels of vitamin E and proteins present in eggs protect the sperm cells against damage from free radicals. If you don't have high blood pressure, or high cholesterol, I would advise you to eat a couple of hardboiled eggs every day. Have one for lunch or breakfast and another for dinner. This will keep your sperm count high all through the day.

Spinach-

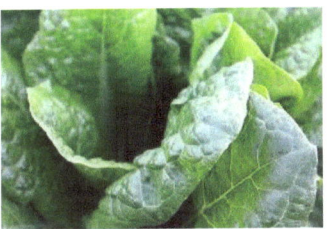

In the above section, we have already discussed about the role played by folic acid in maintaining the health of our sperm. Spinach is one of the richest sources of folic acid. Folic acid deficiency leads to production of malformed sperms. These sperms take a lot of time to reach the egg by penetrating the protective barrier. In addition, low folate levels in the father also increase the chances of birth defects in the baby. Consuming spinach regularly can help in controlling this problem to a great extent. This tip is, however, not for individuals with high levels of uric acid or those suffering from arthritis.

Bananas-

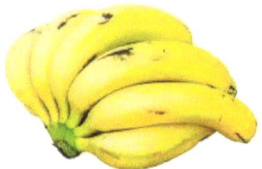

The three main nutrients present in bananas are vitamin C, B1 and A. These nutrients will assist your body to create healthier sperm and will ensure that your sperm count is high. Bananas are rich sources of a rare enzyme known as Bromelain. Bromelain is known for its natural anti-inflammatory qualities and works by boosting sperm count, quality and motility.

Asparagus-

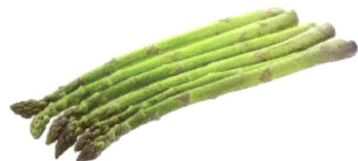

Asparagus is a green vegetable that works by protecting our testicles and fighting free radicals. This boosts sperm production and ensures that all the sperms produced are healthy swimmers. The vitamin C present in asparagus is the primary reason why this vegetable is beneficial in maintaining sperm health.

Broccoli-

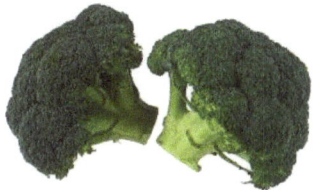

Broccoli is a rich source of vitamin B9 or folic acid. So, it's obvious that this green vegetable would help men in having better sperm count.

Dark chocolates-

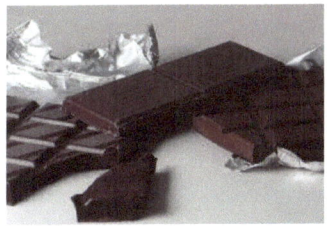

We often associate this food item with lust-filled trysts. You must have seen hotels welcoming couples to their honeymoon suites with a glass of champagne and a bowlful of juicy strawberries dipped in thick, dark chocolate. Many might not know, but there's a hidden reason behind such acts of hotels. Dark chocolate is known for increasing vitality and sperm count dramatically. It's a rich source of L-arginine HCL, an amino acid known both for increasing sperm count and semen volume. That's not all. Some experts say that dark chocolates can also increase the intensity of orgasm.

Pomegranates-

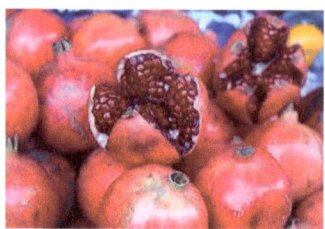

Pomegranates are filled with antioxidants which work by fighting free radicals present in our blood. This ability of the fruit ensures that your sperms are not destroyed by free radicals. Since the ancient times pomegranate juice has been used as a fertility booster.

Garlic-

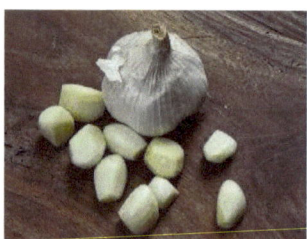

Selenium and vitamin B6 present in garlic enable healthy sperm production. The blood cleaning abilities of garlic are also responsible for making is an amazing fertility booster. Garlic prevents formation of plaques in our arteries and thereby enables improved flow of blood to our testicles. For best results, you should have raw garlic in an empty stomach. If you cannot chew the garlic, mince them and swallow with water.

Walnuts-

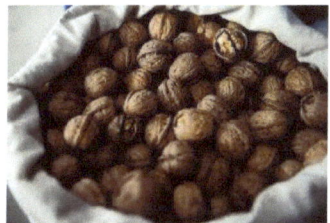

The main active ingredients of walnuts are omega-3 fatty acids, which boost flow of blood to our testicles and increase sperm production. These nuts are also rich in arginine, an agent known for augmenting semen volume. The quantity of antioxidants present in walnuts in two times that of any other type of nut. As a result, these nuts can fight toxins present in the blood stream more efficiently. The less will be the amount of toxins present in your system the better would be the quality of your sperm.

Habits you should avoid for boosting sperm count

There are certain habits that you should let go of when trying to increase your sperm count and semen production. Read on to get acquainted with them.

Keeping your laptop on your lap when working

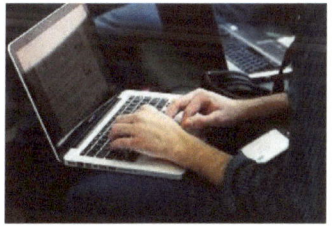

Each one of us must have done this at some point in our lives. It's primarily because the name of the product itself encourages us to do so. If you are a man and still work keeping the laptop on your lap, get rid of the habit today (if you are a woman, stop your partner from doing so immediately). Heat generated from the laptop affects the testicles' temperature directly and decreases the chances of production of healthy sperm. Here, it must be noted that the testicles are located outside out body just to ensure that they remain cool.

Always wearing tight underwear or pants

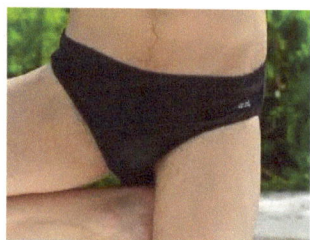

Yes, you have the right of following the latest fashion trends and thereby at times you can surely wear a pair of tight trousers, but doing that always is never recommended. When we wear tight pants or underwear the temperature of our groin area (the region where the scrotum is situated) increases significantly and that's not good for our sperm health.

Overconsumption of alcohol

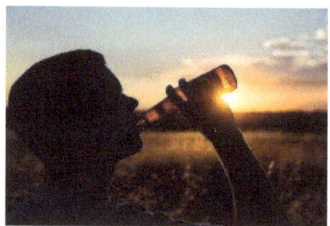

According to a study published recently in the medical journal BMJ Open, men who consume 5 units of alcohol or more per day on a regular basis might experience significant decline in their sperm quality and sperm count.

Applying sunscreen-

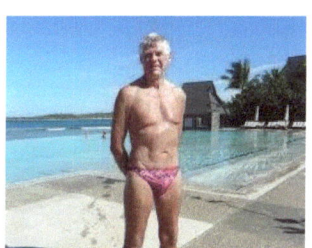

If you want to enjoy being intimate with your partner, I would suggest you to stop taking those sunbaths every weekend. It would not wise to go out in the sun without wearing a sunscreen, but if you do so it will harm the health of your sperm. Findings of a 15-year study revealed that chemicals present in sunscreen lotions and gels and some other cosmetics have direct association with low sperm count and quality. Chemicals such as 3OH-BP or BP-2, which are present in the majority of the sunscreens available on the market, have been found to interfere with male hormones. If you go for a sunbath once in a while, make sure you wash off the sunscreen well after coming back. Wearing it for several hours might destroy your fertility.

Consuming soy in excessive amount

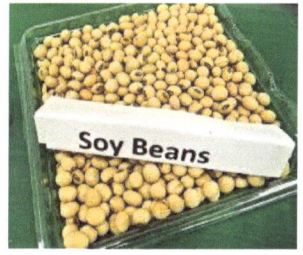

Soy is the most popular source of protein for vegetarians. The isoflavons present in soy make it mimic estrogen in human body. As a result, overconsumption of soy is linked to increase in the levels of female hormone, which can decrease levels of male hormones. So, men should avoid including too much of soy in their daily diet.

Bathing is excessively hot water

Hot baths are truly relaxing. However, if you bath regularly in excessively hot water, it might reduce your sperm count significantly. You should also avoid frequent visits to sauna rooms if you want to have high quality sperm.

Lack of action in bed

Inaction in bed is another habit that can lead to sperm abnormalities. There are instances where men have developed infertility as a result of not having sex for a prolonged period of time. So, to have healthy sperm you must have active sex life.

Smoking

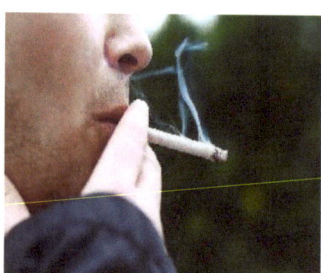

Smoking hampers sperm motility or movement of sperm. Findings of a recent German study revealed that men who smoke regularly experience formation of free radicals in their seminal fluid, which reduces the speed at which sperm moves.

Stress

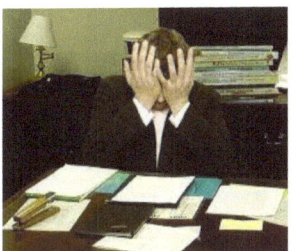

Stress is one of the leading causes of infertility both in men and women. Stress leads to hormonal imbalance in men (and also in women), which affects their sperm health. Practicing meditation, taking part in activities you enjoy etc. can help in relieving stress and getting rid of sperm disorders.

Having a sedentary lifestyle

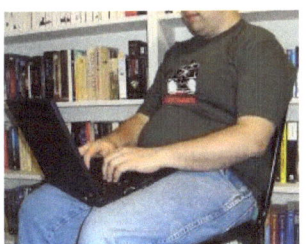

Lack of exercise is a common cause of decline in sperm health and sperm count. Men, who don't work out, tend to have a high BMI (body mass index), which makes them susceptible to a range of health disorders including infertility. Obese men also often have high levels of estrogen, which impairs the process of sperm production. Fat deposits in the groin area can make your testicles non-functional by increasing their temperature.

Conclusion

In this book, I have put together a number of tips and techniques that can help you to rejuvenate your system and experience life extension. You must have noticed that the majority of the suggestions here would require you to change your lifestyle. So, in a nutshell it can be said that to live a life full of vitality, your main target should be having a healthy lifestyle.

Thanks for reading the book!!!

www.ingramcontent.com/pod-product-compliance
Lightning Source LLC
Chambersburg PA
CBHW040914180526
45159CB00010BA/3066